Abdou-Rajack NDIAYE
Sosselem DOLO

The drop

Abdou-Rajack NDIAYE
Sosselem DOLO

The drop

A distinctive phenotype in sub-Saharan Africa

Imprint

Any brand names and product names mentioned in this book are subject to trademark, brand or patent protection and are trademarks or registered trademarks of their respective holders. The use of brand names, product names, common names, trade names, product descriptions etc. even without a particular marking in this work is in no way to be construed to mean that such names may be regarded as unrestricted in respect of trademark and brand protection legislation and could thus be used by anyone.

Cover image: www.ingimage.com

This book is a translation from the original published under ISBN 978-620-6-69422-9.

Publisher:
Sciencia Scripts
is a trademark of
Dodo Books Indian Ocean Ltd. and OmniScriptum S.R.L publishing group

120 High Road, East Finchley, London, N2 9ED, United Kingdom
Str. Armeneasca 28/1, office 1, Chisinau MD-2012, Republic of Moldova, Europe
Printed at: see last page
ISBN: 978-620-6-51735-1

INTRODUCTION

Gout is the most common inflammatory rheumatic disease in males worldwide. It is defined as a microcrystalline arthropathy resulting from the deposition of pro-inflammatory sodium urate microcrystals in tissues. It is the consequence of prolonged hyperuricemia. Hyperuricemia is rarely accompanied by gout. It is defined as a uricemia of over 420 µmol/l (70 mg/l) in men, and over 360 µmol/l (60 mg/l) in women.When urate supersaturation is reached, monosodium urate (MSU) crystals form in the joint. In some individuals, these crystals trigger a self-limiting inflammatory response characteristic of acute gout attacks **[1,2].**

In the 5th century BC, Hippocrates used the word "podagra" to designate gout. This word is at the origin of the French term "podagre", which designates the disease or sufferer of gout. The term was first and foremost descriptive, since in Greek it means "taken by the foot", evoking the trap in which the animal is captured (to designate the foot and agra the hunt or the catch). This counterpart: it was in the 9th century that the term gout was introduced into popular parlance. Rheuma (rheumatism or discharge) is compared to a noxious mood distilled "drop by drop" in the joints as well as the organs. Its meaning narrowed in the 15th century, with the word gout corresponding to the condition known as podagre. In the Renaissance, Ambroise Paré finally adopted the term "gout" in place of podagre. The English used the term "Gout", the Italians "Gotta", the Spanish "Gota" and the Germans "Gicht". The 17th century marked a revolution in the history of rheumatology with the classification of the Parisian physician Guillaume de Baillou, who distinguished gout from other rheumatisms and from what Anglo-Saxons would call arthritis. Descriptions of gout are numerous and long-standing, but one of the most seminal is the treatise on podagre by Thomas Sydenham, nicknamed the English Hippocrates, published in 1683 (Tractatus de Podagra et Hydrope). **[76]**

Gout has also been dubbed "the disease of kings". Indeed, from Charlemagne to

Louis XIV, gout has struck down the great names of history. [77]

Sometimes referred to as an old-fashioned disease, gout was considered in the 19th century to be responsible for all ills (gout remontée). Others saw it as a deserved disease, linked as it was to overeating and debauchery, but also as a benign illness. [78]

Gout is far from being a thing of the past; in fact, it's a rheumatic disease that's on the rise again. In Western Europe, around 5% of the population suffer from gout. These figures are partly linked to the general rise in obesity rates and other genetic and environmental factors. While in the collective imagination, gout is associated with opulence and high-calorie meals, other risk factors come into play. [77]

The prevalence and incidence of gout have been rising steadily over the past forty years. Management of the disease is not always easy, particularly in elderly subjects, due to frequent comorbidities. Few studies have been devoted to gout in Senegal.

EPIDEMIOLOGY

The epidemiological profile of gout has been established in the West by hospital studies and population surveys. Estimates of gout prevalence range from 1 to 1.5%, making it the most common inflammatory arthritis.In the United States, the National Health Interview Survey provides information on the prevalence of gout estimated from self-reporting alone. The prevalence of gout in the general population, measured over the years by this same method, rose from 4.8 ‰ in 1969 to 9.4 ‰ in 1996 for the population as a whole [3]. Recently, analysis of the NHANES (National Health and Nutrition Examination Survey) estimated the prevalence of gout in the USA in the population aged 20 and over at 3.9% in 2007- 2008, whereas it was estimated, in this same database, at 2.7% in the survey conducted from 1988 to 1994, suggesting that the prevalence of the disease continues to rise in the USA [4].

In England, between 1970 and 1990, the prevalence of gout rose from 0.3% to 1% of the total population. Between 2000 and 2005, the gout population rose to 1.4%. This increase in gout prevalence has also affected New Zealand, particularly the Maori, China and Taiwan [5].One of the most important epidemiological studies is the 2005 study by Annemans and associates [6], carried out in Germany and Great Britain. In France, there are no large-scale epidemiological data on gouty disease.This retrospective study of 5 years of data from 2.5 million patients in Great Britain and 2.4 million in Germany showed a prevalence of of gout by 1.4%. Over 80% of gout patients were male. The average age was 66 in Great Britain and 63 in Germany. In Great Britain, the main comorbidity was obesity (27.7%), while in Germany it was diabetes (25.9%). This study has very interesting statistical power. However, it remains retrospective, based on data from general practices. The prevalence between the 2 countries is equivalent, reflecting good reliability of the results obtained. All studies show a very significant increase in the prevalence of gout in recent decades: In New Zealand, prevalence increased almost tenfold in 30 years, from 3/1000 in 1958 to 29/1000 in 1992 in the population of European origin, and almost doubled in the

Maori population, from 27/1000 to 64/1000 (randomized studies) [7-8].

- In the USA, the study by Wallace and associates [9] shows a prevalence that has almost doubled in 10 years, from 2.9/1000 in 1990 to 5.2/1000 in 1999. The study by Lawrence and associates [10] based on the National Health Interviews Surveys (NHIS) shows a prevalence that has almost doubled in 20 years: 4.8/1000 in 1969 and 8.4/1000 in 1992, with a peak prevalence of 9.9/1000 between 1983 and 85.

- In Great Britain, prevalence has increased 7-fold, with a prevalence of 2.3/1000 in 1975 and [11] 14/1000 in 2005[6].A latest study published in January 2015 based on the Clinical Practice Research Datalink (CPRD) estimated the prevalence of gout in Great Britain in 1997 and then in 2012: it rose from 1.52% in 1997 to 2.49% in 2012, a significant increase of 63.9%[12].

In South Africa, the average age is 54.3 for men and 55.3 for women, with a sex ratio of 3.3/1.As for the incidence of gout, various studies show an increase from the 50s to 1990, and a relative stabilization since the 90s/2000s. They also highlight the sex ratio, which clearly favours men, and the fact that the vast majority of gout cases occur in elderly patients.According to the study by Arromde and associates [13], based on the Rochester Epidemiology Project comparing the incidence of gout between 77/78 and 95/96 in the city of Rochester, Minnesota, it increased from 45/100,000 per year to 62.3/100,000 per year. The overall sex ratio between the 2 periods remained stable at 3.3. The incidence of primary gout increased more than 2-fold between the 2 periods, with statistical significance (p=0.002).The study by Kuo and associates [12], analyzing CPRD data from the UK, showed an incidence of gout of 1.36/1000 per year in 1997 and 1.77/1000 per year in 2012, an increase of 29.6%. The overall sex ratio fell from 3.4 to 3. This reflects an increase in incidence in the female population. The study by Elliot, based on data from the Royal College of General Practitioners between 1994 and 2007, shows a stable incidence of gout over this period in both men and women. [14]

PATHOPHYSIOLOGY

II.1 Hyperuricemia

Hyperuricemia is defined by the serum uric acid concentration above which there is a risk of gout: this is 360 µmol/l in men and women according to the European League Against Rheumatism (EULAR) [15]. The risk of symptomatic disease increases with persistent hyperuricemia.Uric acid is the end product of purine metabolism in humans, who have lost the uricase required to oxidize it to allantoin during evolution [16]. There are 3 mechanisms of uric acid entry: de novo purinosynthesis, catabolism of cellular nucleic acids and catabolism of dietary nucleic acids:

- **De novo purinosynthesis**

The purine nucleus is entirely elaborated, essentially in the liver, from fragments of simple molecules abundantly available in the body (bicarbonate and amino acids including glutamine). These "precursors" bind to phospho-ribosyl-pyrophosphate (PRPP), which acts as a ribose-phosphate donor. PRPP, in turn, is formed from ATP and ribose 5-phosphate by phospho-ribosyl synthetase. In the first stage, glutamine is bound to PRPP to form phospho-ribosylamine (PRA), under the action of a specific aminotransferase. This first step is irreversible. The purine nucleus is then formed in successive stages. It always carries the original ribose phosphate. So the first stage doesn't result in a purine base, but in a nucleotide: inosinic acid (IMP). This is the hub of purine metabolism, and is transformed into AMP and GMP, which are incorporated into complex nucleic acid molecules. [79]

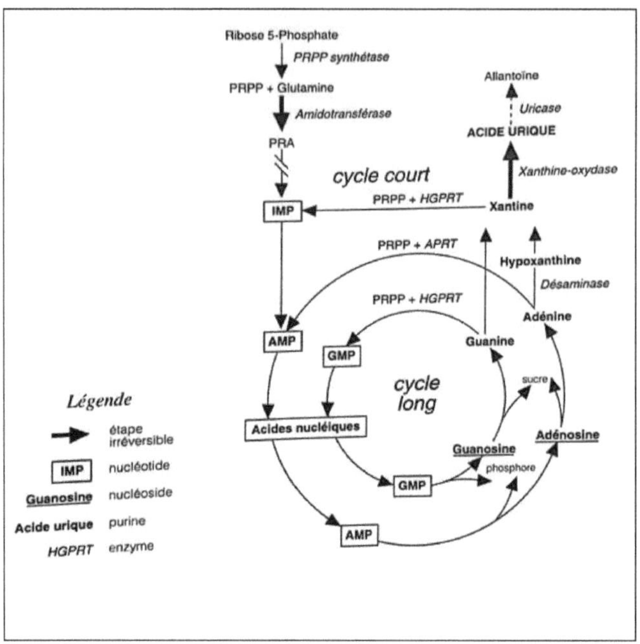

Figure 1: Diagram of uric acid metabolism

•Catabolism of endogenous nucleic acids

This is the catabolism of cellular nucleic acids. Like all the body's proteins, these nucleic acids are constantly being renewed.They are then broken down into purine nucleotides, then nucleosides and finally purine bases, which can either be transformed into uric acids or reused for new nucleotide synthesis, which is much less energetically costly than de novo synthesis. This completes the cycle The long metabolic cycle is referred to as the "long" cycle, as opposed to the "short" cycle, which goes directly from the nucleotides resulting from de novo synthesis to the purine bases. The long cycle is quantitatively the most important under normal conditions in terms of uric acid production.

•Catabolism of exogenous (dietary) nucleic acids

Generally speaking, all proteins are "purinogenic", but certain "purinophoric" foods are particularly rich in nucleoproteins. After successive digestive degradation, the purine bases released can be used to build new nucleotides, or transformed into uric acid by oxidative deamination. In this way, guanine produces xanthine, while adenosine produces hypoxanthine. Hypoxanthine is transformed into xanthine and xanthine into uric acid. These last two steps are carried out by xanthine oxidase, the enzyme inhibited by allopurinol. Uric acid is the ultimate end of catabolism in humans because it lacks the uricase enzyme which enables it to be broken down into allantoin. **[79]**

• **Regulation of purinosynthesis**

Nucleotide synthesis is essentially negative feedback on amidotranferase: the rate of nucleotide synthesis regulates de novo synthesis according to need. These nucleotides may come directly from this purinosynthesis, but also from the recombination of a purine base with PRPP thanks to hypoxanthine-guanine-phosphoribosyl-tranferase (HGPRT) or adenine-phospho-ribosyl-tranferase (APRT), depending on the purine base[79].

• **Uric acid elimination**

- Uricolysis

Digestive uricolysis involves twenty to twenty-five percent of uric acid. This proportion of uric acid is discharged into the intestine by secretions digestive tract. Intestinal bacteria, equipped with uricases, then degrade the uric acid into allantoin, which is eliminated via the fecal route. Intra-tissular uricolysis is also possible, but the amount is negligible.

- **Renal elimination**

Free uric acid levels (uraturia) average 750mg/d (4414 μmol). Uric acid clearance is 8mg/min (0.13mg/s). In urine, uric acid is ionized and urates are present in variable proportions according to pH. The more basic the pH, the more the equilibrium shifts towards the bound form. This bound form is 17 times more soluble than the ionized form. Urinary acidity favors uric lithiasis, as the less-soluble ionized form increases to the detriment of the more-soluble bound form.

Glomerular filtration is classically estimated at 95% of plasma uric acid. Tubular resorption is authenticated by the fact that uric acid clearance is much lower than creatinine clearance. This resorption takes place in the proximal tubule via an active transport mechanism. Tubular secretion is also evidenced by the existence of hypouricemia, with the ratio of uric acid clearance to creatinine clearance greater than 1. This tubular secretion explains the inverse effects of certain drugs, depending on the dosage used (Aspirin, Phenylbutazone, Probenecid): at low doses, these drugs reduce tibular secretion, thus decreasing uraturia by reducing uric acid resorption[79].

- **Mechanisms of hyperuricemia**

Hyperuricemia is a biological anomaly characterized by an abnormally high level of circulating uric acid in the blood, which on its own does not indicate disease. However, hyperuricemia is a necessary or at least sufficient condition for the onset of gout. This hyperuricemia is defined by a blood level of blood uric acid above 70mg/l (412 µmol/l). the reasons are as follows:

-Biochemical reason: limits saturation of uric acid in plasma

-Clinical reason: uric acid levels in gout sufferers are almost always 70 mg/l or higher.

-Statistical reason: as the limit of the standard is defined as the mean ± 2 standard deviations, values close to 70 mg/l are again obtained with the uricase enzymatic assay. [79]

II.2 Gouty access

Neutrophils and monocytes/macrophages are the main cellular players in the acute microcrystalline inflammatory reaction. The acute attack is triggered as follows: The inflammatory reaction in the joints is triggered by the presence of sodium urate microcrystals (UMS) in the joint cavity [17]. These crystals infiltrate the synovium and are released into the synovial cavity.

It consists of several phases [18] [19] (see Figure 2):

1) Intra-articular irruption of crystals from cartilage or synovial deposits;

2) Activation phase of synovial membrane cells and production of pro-inflammatory cytokines and chemokines;

3) Stimulation phase of capillary endothelial cells and mast cells ;

4) Synovial recruitment phase of blood monocytes and articular PNN ;

5) Amplification phase of the reaction followed by **(6)** Spontaneous Resolution **[20]**.

Microcrystals can activate cells in two ways:

- Phagocytosis of UMS crystals by macrophages and then PNNs, inducing release of lysosomal enzymes and activation of pro-inflammatory cytokines.

- By direct interaction between cells and bare, non-protein-coated crystals (electrostatic binding or direct binding to a membrane receptor) or protein-coated crystals (protein adsorbed on the crystal surface, such as CD14, then activating signalling pathways such as G proteins, Src tyrosine kinases, etc.) **[21]**.

• Inflammasome and initiation of the inflammatory response:

Interleukin-1β and the Inflammasome play a key role in gouty access **[22, 23]**. The production and activation of Interlekin-1β occurs in three steps:

1) NOD-like receptors (mainly NALP3) form the Inflammasome complex. The presence of UMS crystals leads to the formation of the Inflammasome, inducing caspase-1 activation. Activated caspase-1 induces the production of Interleukin-1ß precursor **[23]**.

2) Production of a pro-Il-1β precursor through Nf-kB action (Nuclear Factor KappaB, a transcription family protein involved in the immune response).

- This pr-Il-1β precursor undergoes maturation to give Il-1β thanks to caspase-1, which was already activated by the Inflammasome. This interleukin-1β is the main enzyme.

- Amplification of the inflammatory reaction :

Once inflammation is triggered by Il-1β, blood monocytes and resident mast cells are the first cells activated in the inflammation chain [**18, 19**]. They secrete histamine, inflammatory cytokines (TNFα and Il-1β) and other Il-1β. They activate endothelial cells and promote PNN recruitment. Intra-articular PNN are attracted by a chemotactic gradient (C5a and Il-8). PNN-crystal interaction and phagocytosis are responsible for the amplification of the inflammatory phenomenon.

- Spontaneous resolution of acute inflammation :

Macrophages and monocytes are the cells that regulate the inflammatory response. Depending on their state of differentiation, phagocytes can tip the balance from an asymptomatic state to acute inflammation, and vice versa [**18**] [**19**]. This change of state or monocyte/macrophage "switch" is accompanied by a loss of capacity to produce pro-inflammatory cytokines (IL-1, IL-6, TNF-α) and d conversely, to gain the ability to secrete anti-inflammatory cytokines (IL-10, TGF-β) after phagocytosing UMS crystals [**20**].

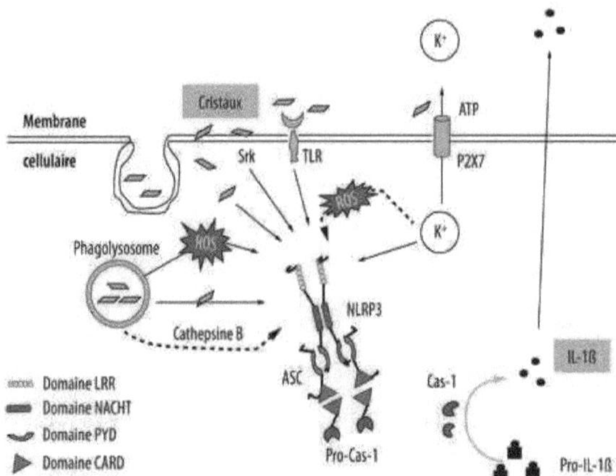

Figure 2: Chain of inflammatory activation during a gouty attack

II.3 Chronic inflammation and chondrocyte activation

Gouty arthropathy with intra- and periarticular tophus develops after years of untreated hyperuricemia. The tophus is surrounded by a granulomatous reaction, leading to chronic synovitis and destruction of bone and cartilage.The presence of monocytes at different stages of evolution has been identified: recently migrated monocytes around vessels, resident macrophages organized in granulomas. They express TNF-α and metallo proteases (MMP-2 and MMP-9) [24]. Dalbeth et al described CD 68+ macrophages expressing Il-1 and TGF-1 in the first ring of cells surrounding the tophus [25]. This suggests that tophus actively contributes to a cycle of chronic inflammation, overwhelmed by its attempts at access resolution and tissue repair.Researchers have also speculated that additional pathophysiological pathways are activated: activation of osteoclastogenesis (bone destruction) [25], inhibition of osteoblast activity [26, 27], link between chronic inflammation proportional to tophaceous mass and development of atherosclerosis.

IDENTIFICATION OF FACTORS OF RISK FACTORS AND COMORBIDITIES OF GOUT

III.1 Genetic factors

Recent years have seen considerable advances in our understanding of the genetic basis of hyperuricemia and gout, and we now have sufficient information on the genes identified as important in the onset of hyperuricemia.In a recent study of American male twins, the authors found no difference in the prevalence of gout between monozygotic and dizygotic twins. However, monozygotic twins were twice as likely to have hyperuricemia as dizygotic twins (53% vs. 24%).

%). These results led the authors of the study to conclude that hyperuricemia was genetically determined, while the development of gout was linked to environmental factors.Most of the genes identified are involved in either urate excretion or reabsorption in the renal tubule [30].

The SLC22A12 gene encodes the URAT1 (Human Urat transporter 1) protein, which acts in concert with other transporters. This gene is important in controlling uric acid reabsorption in the proximal renal tubule. A polymorphism in this gene has been associated with under-excretion of uric acid and hyperuricemia in Caucasian Germans [31].

Concerning the SLC2A9 gene encoding the GLUT9 protein, which is a transporter of glucose and fructose, but also of uric acid in the proximal renal tubule, the association between a polymorphism of SLC2A9 and hyper uricemia or gout was confirmed in a study comparing whole genomes in 3 cohorts [32].

The study also identified 2 associated genes, ABCG2 (an efflux transporter of uric acid in collecting tubule cells) and SLC17A3 (encoding NPT4, a Na/P co-transporter in the proximal tubule). The discovery of these genes and the influence of their polymorphism on uric acid levels could make it possible to establish a probability score for the onset of gout.Research into genetic susceptibility in gout is interesting, but remains difficult to dissociate in the elderly, due to the presence of numerous comorbidities (dietary, iatrogenic, renal aging), and studies on the genetics of hyperuricemia must be clearly targeted at young subjects, without comorbidity.

III.2 Hyperuricemia

Hyperuricemia has been identified as the most important risk factor in the development of gout.The risk of gout increases with the degree and duration of hyperuricemia, and the frequency of attacks increases exponentially for uricemia above 420 µmol/l. Thus, in a prospective 15-year study of 2,000 men, the annual incidence of gout rose from 0.01% for uraemia below 420µmol/l, to 0.09% for uraemia between 420 and 480 µmol/l, and to 4.9% when uraemia exceeded 540 µmol/l [28].

However, it should be remembered that only 10% of hyperuricemic subjects will develop gout, suggesting other, as yet unknown, factors in the onset of this disease.Hyperuricemia, in turn, is favored by other factors such as the use of drugs like diuretics and renal failure, which is why it is frequently associated with other metabolic disorders [29].

III.3 Alcohol consumption

The ingestion of strong alcohols, beer with or without alcohol, and sodas rich in fructose sometimes significantly increases uricemia. Beers are rich in purines, including alcohol-free beers, which contain guanosine [28].

However, the level of risk varies according to the different alcohols, being lower with wine and higher with guanosine-rich beer than with strong spirits. Virtually all studies have shown that alcohol consumption increases the prevalence and incidence of gout. For example, in the Framingham cohort, the incidence of gout was 3 times higher in women and 2 times higher in men for pure alcohol consumption exceeding 207 ml per week. The relative risk of gout in men, in the American Health Professionals Follow-up Study, rose from 1.32 for alcohol consumption of 10 to 15 g/d, to 2.53 for consumption of over 50 g/d, particularly for beer (355 ml/d) and strong spirits (44 ml/d); there was no increase in risk with wine (118 ml) **[33]**.

III.4 Medicines

Several drugs are regularly incriminated in so-called medicated gout. Foremost among these are diuretics and cyclosporine. Others, such as low-dose acetylsalicylic acid (AA), can cause hyperuricemia. Other molecules play a more anecdotal role. The list of these drugs is summarized in **Table I [34]**.

Table I: Drugs inducing hyperuricemia **[34].**

Drug name	Hyperuricemia	The drop
Diuretics	+	+
B-blockers	+	-
Acetylsalicylic acid (low dose)	+	-
Ciclosporin	+	+
Tacrolimus	+	+
Pyrazinamide	+	+/-
Ethambutol	+	+/-
Ritonavir	+	+

III.5 Renal insufficiency

Various forms of kidney disease can impair urinary uric acid elimination. But chronic kidney disease is the main cause of secondary hyperuricemia.
It comes in two forms:

-Renal lithiasis

Urolithiasis is present in 20-40% of gout sufferers, but can also occur in subjects with no joint manifestations whatsoever. Two essential factors are involved in the genesis of uric lithiasis: hyperuraturia > 600 mg/24h, and above all urinary hyperacidity, which is constant in gouty patients.

-Gout nephropathy

This is found in 10-20% of chronic gout sufferers. It is a chronic interstitial nephropathy which may be the consequence of lithiasis or due to precipitation of urate crystals in the renal medulla. **[79]**

III.6 **Metabolic syndrome**

Gout was originally part of the metabolic syndrome. A strong association was found between metabolic syndrome and gout: a study using data from the Third National Health and Nutrition Examination Survey, conducted between 1988 and 1994, compared the prevalence of metabolic syndrome (defined using National Cholesterol Education Program Adult Treatment Panel III criteria) in subjects with gout with controlled subjects without gout. Among gout sufferers, 62.8% had a metabolic syndrome, compared with 25.4% in gout-free subjects (OR=3.05 2.01-4.61 IC 95%) **[35]**.

CLINICAL EXPRESSION OF GOUT

The drop is classically described in 3 stages : asymptomatic hyperuricemia, acute gout and chronic gout or tophacea.Diagnostic criteria are straightforward: acute attack involving the big toe, notion of lithiasis and family history, progressive course of the attack with or without treatment.In the chronic stage, the presence of tophus is characteristic. Examination of sodium urate synovial fluid is of great interest. It can be used to identify highly birefringent intra- or extracellular sodium urate crystals with pointed ends. These crystals are dissolved by urikinase. They should be preserved in a hydroalcoholic solution after puncture. [79]

IV.1 Acute gout

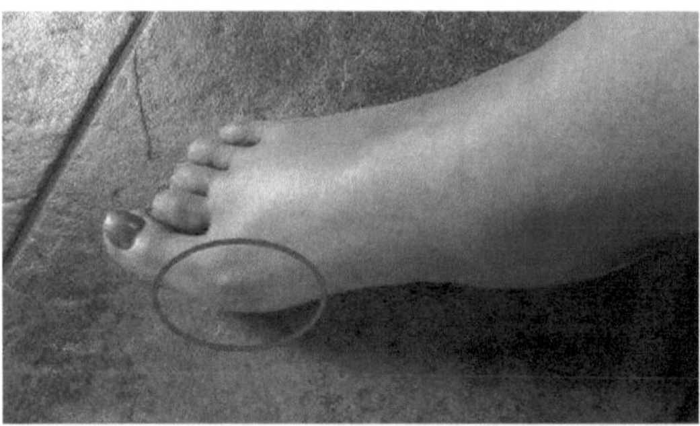

Figure 3: Gout attack (arthritis of the first metatarsophalangeal joint with swollen joint, hyperesthetic shiny skin)

It generally occurs after a triggering factor such as excessive eating or drinking, trauma or medication. This crisis may be preceded by prodromal symptoms such as malaise, irritability or local tingling paresthesias.Gout attacks often occur at night. It is often rapid, lasting between 6 and 12 hours on average. Intense, violent pain, generally mono-articular (85%). There is an inflammatory stigma in the affected joint, with intense swelling, associated with local heat and marked erythema. Pain is most intense during the 2nd half of the night. This is why it's known as "crowing" pain, aggravated by contact with the bed sheet, due to significant cutaneous hyperesthesia.General inflammatory signs are mainly characterized by fever, which can reach 39°C **[15]**.

Generally, the first attack affects the lower limb (85-90% of cases). The first attack classically involves the first metatarsophalangeal joint **[36]**.

Progression is spontaneously favorable within 5 to 10 days. A good response after 48 hours of treatment is an additional diagnostic factor. In the elderly, gout tends to affect the distal interphalangeal joints of the fingers, already affected by osteoarthritis. It is also more often polyarticular.In terms of evolution, 60% of patients will suffer a new attack within a year of the first. Recurrences of gouty attacks may be oligo or even polyarticular, with a topography that frequently extends to the upper limbs, particularly the hands and wrists. These attacks may be extra-articular, taking the form of olecranon or pre-patellar bursitis, tendonitis or tenosynovitis. In the medium to long term, gouty attacks tend to become less frank but increasingly prolonged, with shorter and shorter free intervals.

Table II: Diagnostic criteria (EULAR 2006)

Recommendations for diagnosing gout

• *A gout attack is characterized by severe pain, swelling, and tenderness that reaches its peak in 6-12 hours, with a suggestive but non-specific erythema.*

• *In the case of a typical presentation, clinical diagnosis alone is possible, but not definitive in the absence of confirmation of crystals.*

• *The demonstration of urate crystals in the fluid or a tophus provides a definite diagnosis.*

• *A test for microcrystals is recommended on any joint fluid from undifferentiated arthritis.*

• *The identification of crystals in an asymptomatic joint can lead to a diagnosis in an inter-critical period.*

• *Gout and septic arthritis may coexist, warranting direct examination and culture if infection is suspected even in the presence of microcrystals.*

• Uricemia does not confirm or exclude a gout attack, as some hyperuricemic patients never have a gout attack, and some patients have normal uricemia during a gout attack.

• Uraturia should be evaluated in certain patients, particularly in cases of family history, early onset or renal calculi.

• Although X-rays are useful for differential diagnosis and can show typical aspects of chronic gout, they are not useful for confirming acute or recent gout.

• Risk factors for gout and associated comorbidities must be assessed, including metabolic syndrome (obesity, hyperglycemia, hyperlipidemia and hypertension).

IV.2 Clinical forms

IV.2.1 Symptomatic forms

- Acute gouty attack:

The attack may take on a pseudo-phlegmoneous form, leading to unnecessary surgery. In such cases, the patient's history, the existence of tophus, the isolated nature of the condition and its good tolerance are all important factors.

- Mild access :

This is the asthenic form, either spontaneously or due to inadequate treatment. The heat is bearable, the swelling moderate, but generally lasts longer, leaving some discrete stiffness.

IV.2.2 Topographic shapes :

Unusually, gout may also affect another joint. In order of frequency, these include the medio-tarsal, the ankle, the calcaneo-thalian, the knee, the wrist, the finger and the elbow. Other joints have also been reported, including the shoulder and sternoclavicular joint. Para-articular localizations such as Achilles tendonitis, crow's-foot tendonitis, acute plantar talalgia or retro-olecranial and pre-patellar bursitis are easily identifiable, as they are often accompanied by a typical crisis, or have the characteristics of a crisis. Other forms described that are more difficult to relate to gout are superficial phlebitis, pharyngitis, laryngitis, parotitis, orchitis, pericarditis, conjunctivitis and gouty iritis.

•Oligo or acute gouty arthritis:

Forms affecting several joints have been described, particularly in the elderly (>60 years) and in secondary drops.

•Spinal topography

Spinal topography is characterized by axial involvement, with often lumbar, inflammatory spinal pain coexisting with tophi around the spinal zone.

IV.2.3 Early drop :

The onset of gout in young men or premenopausal women should raise the rare possibility of an enzymatic abnormality leading to increased uric acid production. This early-onset gout may take the form of renal lithiasis, neurological disorders or familial uratic nephropathy.The gene corresponding to this nephropathy has been located on the short arm of chromosome 16.The enzymatic mechanisms involved in uric acid hyperproduction are either a deficiency of HGPRT, glucose-6-phosphate or fructose-1-phosphate aldolase; or, on the contrary, hyperactivity of PRPP.These mechanisms reflect rare anomalies. However, in heterozygosity deficiency, the prevalence of fructose-1-phosphate aldolase is 1/250.In this heterozygous group, one in three people will develop gout. For this reason, heterozygosity is a frequent cause of familial gout in frustose-1-phosphate deficiency. **[81]**

IV.2.4 Female drop:

Rare before the menopause, it is more common in the elderly, notably due to the co-prescription of diuretics. In elderly women, it is characterized by tophi localized on the fingers without arthropathy, or by digital osteoarthritis lesions. [85]

IV.2.5 Secondary drop :

Secondary forms of gout occur when dyspurinemia is linked to a specific cause. We distinguish :

- Hemopathy due to cell lysis. This is the case with polycythemia gout, leukemia, myeloma, lymphoma and solid tumors treated with cytolytic agents.
- Global renal failure due to nephropathy of any kind.

Hyperuricemia is common in renal failure, and may eventually lead to gout, particularly in long-standing nephropathies such as polycystic kidney disease;
- Lead poisoning, with a renal and haematological mechanism

- Diuretics: thiazides, furosemide and etacrinic acid

- Antituberculosis drugs: Pyrazinamide and Ethambutol, which frequently increase uricemia.
- Low-dose aspirin;

- Conditions such as myxedema, hyperparathyroidism, psoriasis, sarcoidosis, beryllium intoxication and diabetic acidosis, in which transplantation followed by ciclosporin prescription can lead to asymptomatic hyperuricemia. Gout is a frequent (10-20% of cases) and serious complication. It occurs after organ transplantation. It is characterized by its early onset, its severity, the short time between symptomatic gout and hyperuricemia. [84]

IV.3   Chronic gout

Chronic gout sets in after about ten years of evolution. It is characterized, on the one hand, by chronic polyarticular involvement and, on the other, by the appearance of tophus. In the absence of treatment, tophaceous gout sets in within 5 years of the onset of the disease. This is the case in 30% of patients [36].

Polyarticular involvement is manifested by persistent acute synovitis, symmetrical or not, typically sparing hips and shoulders. At this stage of the disease, gouty arthropathy develops. All joints, and exceptionally the spine, may be affected [37].

The appearance of tophus is characteristic of chronic gout. These are white deposits, organized into painless nodules. They vary in size, and are found preferentially in the auricle, periarticular areas, particularly in the hands, and in the bursae of the olecranon, prepatellar and tendon structures (primarily the Achilles tendon). Subcutaneous tophus can be found in extra-articular locations on the legs and forearms, and to a lesser extent on the buttocks, thighs and abdominal wall. These locations are indicative of a highly advanced disease.

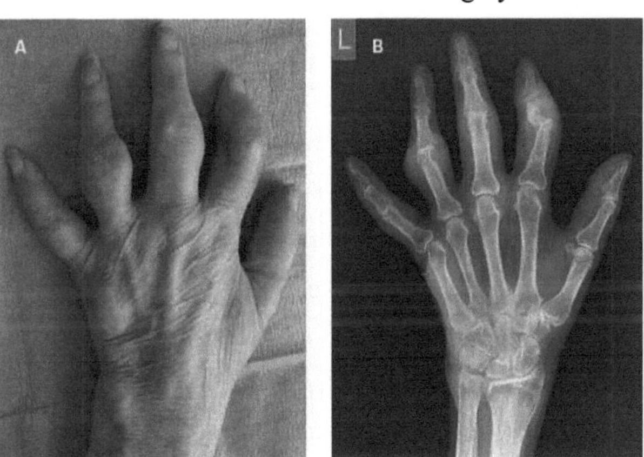

Figure 4: Microcrystalline arthropathy [86]

FURTHER TESTS [80-83]

V.1 Biological examination

Blood tests (CBC) may show an increase in leukocytes (hyperleukocytosis), VS and CRP.Uricemia is frequently normal (30%) during acute attacks, hence the need to measure it at a distance from the attack.The definitive diagnosis of gout is based on the direct identification of monosodium urate crystals in synovial fluid, and the exclusion of septic arthritis. Joint fluid should therefore be punctured with aseptic technique. Synovial fluid is inflammatory, with a predominance of neutrophils. Monosodium urate crystals, intracellular or extracellular, are visible under a polarized light microscope, as negatively birefringent crystals. 24-hour uraturia, a fundamental element in therapy, must be measured.Renal function (creatinine level and clearance) should be systematically investigated. Look for hypertension and metabolic disorders associated with hyperuricemia (hypercholesterolemia, hypertriglyceridemia, hyperglycemia).

V.2 Radiological images [69]

During the initial acute attack, the only radiological sign is a swelling with thickening of the periarticular soft tissues, which is totally specific. In the late chronic phase, the changes induced are highly polymorphic and include :

- Soft particle swellings resulting from chronic metabolic deposits, which are tophi.

- Cartilage may be the site of urea deposits. Occasionally, gout may manifest itself as atypical osteoarthritis, with a destructive tendency and little reconstruction (few osteophytes). This situation is rare, as in the majority of cases, cartilage damage is minimal. Relatively normal joint spaces, in the case of largely erosive arthropathies, are a good argument in favour of gouty disease.

- Bone erosions are the most typical radiological feature:

o Erosions are most often asymmetrical marginal, juxta or para-articular, or even located at a distance from the joints.

o Typically, these are circumscribed (cookie-cutter) erosions with a geodic appearance.

o Chronic erosions tend to present raised bone margins, suggesting a progressive increase in intra-osseous tophi. Uplift of the cortex, inducing focal periosteal neoformation, determines very characteristic erosions, with overhanging margins.

o Para-articular erosions with marginal bone spicules on the surface of the tarsus can create a rather unusual appearance: the spiky gouty foot.

o In some cases, juxta or para-articular tophic expansions can be voluminous, resulting in mutilating arthritis, or take on a quasi-tumoral appearance, even leading to complete amputation of the phalanges.

TREATMENT

The most common treatments for gout have long been known, but in some cases they have become problematic or even contraindicated, making the management of this pathology complicated, particularly in the poly-pathological elderly. In cases where conventional treatment is not possible, practitioners have recently been offered other therapeutic options, some of which are still undergoing trials. We will first discuss the treatment of the acute gout attack, followed by treatments to reduce uricemia levels based on the American College of Rheumatology (ACR) recommendations published in 2012 and recent clinical research data [38,39].

VI.1 Goals [76]

- Soothe the pain of gout attacks;

- Reduce uric acid levels in the blood (use of hypo-uricemics);

- Prevent recurrence of gout attacks.

VI.2 Resources
VI.2.1 Crisis treatment

The main aim of gout attack treatment is to provide pain relief, which must be obtained rapidly. According to ACR recommendations (figure 2), management is based on the following elements:

- Treatment is medicated.

- It is initiated early, within 24 hours of the onset of the seizure.

- Urea-lowering treatment should be continued during the crisis.

- Patient education must be carried out so that they can start treatment before consulting a doctor in the future.

Drug treatment is chosen according to pain intensity (from mild/moderate with VAS $\leq$ 6 to severe VAS>6) and the number of joints affected (1 or 2 large joints or a few small ones and more than 4 joints).

For mild to moderate seizures, the ACR recommends three treatment options:

- Non-steroidal anti-inflammatory drugs (NSAIDs),

- -Systemic corticoids systemic corticoids,

- Oral colchicine.

In the event of a severe seizure, a combination of :

- Colchicine and NSAIDs,

- Oral corticosteroids and colchicine,

- Intra-articular corticosteroids and one of the above treatments.

No classification between drugs has been proposed. This leaves the choice of initial treatment to the doctor.The expected efficacy of the chosen medication, the results of this or that treatment in previous attacks, and the patient's comorbidities.

VI.2.1.1 Drug treatment

•Non-steroidal anti-inflammatory drugs

The ACR responded in the same way as the Food and Drug Association (FDA) and the European Medical Agency, recommending full-dose NSAIDs for gout attacks. NSAIDs, which inhibit prostaglandin-2 and cyclooxygenase production, should be used with caution in cases of arterial hypertension, cardiac, coronary, hepatic or renal insufficiency, and in the elderly **[40, 41]**. Contraindications include active peptic ulcer disease (PUD), severe renal or hepatic insufficiency, and drug combinations such as anticoagulants, lithium, digoxin and diuretics. The molecules approved by the FDA for the treatment of gout are naproxen, indomethacin and sulindac. They are initiated and continued at full dose until the attack is completely cured.With regard to cyclooxygenase-2 inhibitors, in cases of intolerance to conventional NSAIDs and/or digestive contraindications, randomized trials show the efficacy of etoricoxib [43] and lumiracoxib [44]. Lumiracoxib is not marketed due to its high hepatotoxicity. A comparative study of celecoxib versus indomethacin [45] demonstrated the efficacy of celecoxib at high doses (800 mg in 1 dose on day [1], then 400 mg the same day and 400 mg twice a day for 7 days). The ACR recommends celecoxib as a 2nd-line treatment in cases of intolerance or contraindication to conventional NSAIDs [39].

• **Colchicine**

Colchicine, a tricyclic alkaloid extracted from autumn colchicum (Colchicum autumnale), has been used for over 2,000 years to treat gout attacks [46]. Its main mechanism of action is based on inhibition of cytoskeletal microtubule polymerization by binding to β-tubulin, preventing the function and inhibition of IL 1β production and activity [47, 48]. In France, colchicine remains the reference treatment for gout attacks. It is also used as a therapeutic test.Like NSAIDs, colchicine is recommended by EULAR as a first-line treatment, but only within the first 36 hours of the onset of the attack [27].

The ACR recommends the following scheme:

- a loading dose of 1.2 mg (or 1 mg if 0.5 mg tablets only are available)
- then 0.6 mg (or 0.5 mg) one hour later,

- 0.6 mg 12 hours later, once or twice a day (or 0.5 mg twice or three times a day) until crisis resolution [39].

Because of its digestive toxicity, the current trend is to reduce doses. The British Society of Rheumatology (BSR) and EULAR recommend low doses: 0.5 mg three times a day [42, 27].

In cases of mild renal impairment (clearance between 50 and 80 ml/min) or moderate renal impairment (clearance between 30 and 50 ml/min). No dose adjustment is necessary. However, close monitoring is necessary to avoid possible side effects. In cases of severe renal insufficiency (cl<30 ml/min), treatment should not be repeated more than once every 2 weeks, without the need for dose adjustment.

In patients requiring frequent treatment, it is preferable to choose another therapeutic option (FDA recommendations).

•Systemic and intra-articular corticoids

Corticosteroids, anti-inflammatory agents derived from synthetic glucocorticoids, are the natural choice when NSAIDs and colchicine are contraindicated **[49, 50]**. This situation is relatively common in the multi-pathological elderly.

Oral corticosteroids are recommended by the ACR if one or two joints are affected. If one or two large joints are involved, the ACR also recommends intra-articular corticosteroids, the dosage of which is based on the size of the joint.

If intra-articular injection is not possible (polyarticular involvement, patient choice, or joint difficult to inject), oral corticosteroids (prednisone or prednisolone) are recommended at a dose of at least 0.5 mg / kg per day for 5 to 10 days. Or 2 to 5 days at full dose, then 7 to 10 days at decreasing dose.

•Therapeutic combinations

In the event of a severe attack (VAS ≥ 7), or if the attack is polyarticular or involves a large joint, combination therapy is recommended up to the full dose. Response may be incomplete despite initial treatment. In this case, the ACR expert committee defines inadequate pain relief as a reduction in VAS of less than 20% on the first day. In such cases, it is recommended to reconsider the diagnosis first, and then either to change treatment among those proposed, or to add a molecule.In the case of an incomplete response despite initial treatment, the ACR expert committee defines as insufficient pain relief (measured by a VAS) the following cases:

- less than 20% in the first 24 hours

- or less than 50% after 24 hours of treatment initiation. In either of these cases, it is advisable to reconsider the diagnosis first, and then either change the proposed treatment or add another molecule.

•New treatments for gouty arthritis: IL-1β inhibitors

Evidence of a major role for the inflammasome and interleukin 1β (IL-1β) in the development of acute gouty attacks prompted an evaluation of the efficacy of IL-1β inhibitors in the treatment of gouty attacks. Their mechanism is explained in figure5.

Three compounds have shown encouraging results: anakinra (Il-1Ra), rilonacept (Il1-Trap) and canakinumab. Anakinra is a recombinant receptor inhibitor. Rilonacept is a fusion protein of the soluble Il-1 receptor.Canakinumab is an anti-Il-1β monoclonal antibody.Anakinra does not yet have marketing authorization for gout attacks. Rilonacept is no longer marketed in France. Canakinumab is indicated for severe gouty arthritis (more than 3 episodes per year) refractory to or contraindicated by conventional therapies, at a dose of 150 mg subcutaneous injection, which may be administered as a single dose. repeated at intervals of at least 12 weeks. It should be administered as soon as possible after the onset of an attack.For Il-1 antagonism to be maximally effective in the treatment of gout attacks, it should be introduced very early to halt the effects of the Il-1 cascade, ideally before other cytokines are released. On the other hand, prophylaxis with an Il-1 antagonist at the time of initiation of hypouricemic therapy, in the absence of active gout, is theoretically more interesting and potentially highly effective. Il-1 inhibitors appear to have a place in the preventive treatment of gout attacks following the introduction of hypo-uremic therapy, as shown by two recent studies.A first study [51] evaluated canakinumab in 432 patients starting allopurinol therapy. They were divided into 7 different treatment groups: one taking colchicine at a dose of 0.5 mg/d for 16 weeks (control), and the other 6 receiving different doses of canakinumab in a single subcutaneous injection (only one "monthly" group received 3 doses of canakinumab, 50 mg on d1 and 25 mg on d57 and d85). At the end of the study, the percentage of patients having had at least one gout attack during the 16 weeks varied from 14.8 to 27.3 in the canakinumab groups versus 44.4 in the colchicine group (p < 0.05). Multiple injections did not improve efficacy. The percentage of adverse events was similar in all groups.A second PRE-SURGE study [52] was conducted with rilonacept, in 241 patients with multiple annual gout attacks and chronic hyperuricemia, starting on allopurinol 300 mg/d, followed for 16 weeks. Patients were divided into 3 groups: a placebo group, a weekly subcutaneous rilonacept 80 mg group and a weekly subcutaneous rilonacept 160 mg group.Patients receive a double dose of rilonacept (160 or 320 mg) on Day 1, and then return to the normal dose the following week.Gout attacks were significantly reduced in the 2 rilonacept groups compared with the placebo group.The percentage of patients with at least one gout attack at S16 was 46.8% in the placebo group, versus 18.8% and 16.3% respectively in the rilonacept 80 and 160 mg groups (p <0.005). There was no difference in the occurrence of severe adverse events between the 3 groups.

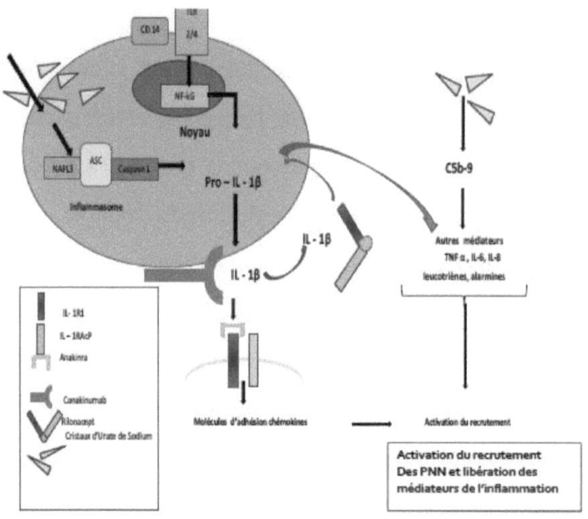

Figure 4: IL-1β inhibitor action diagram

VI.2.1.2 Non-drug treatments :

The ACR expert committee has recommended the use of ice on painful joints [39].

VI.2.2 Background treatment

Hyperuricemia, defined as an elevation of serum uric acid above 360 µmol/l in men and women, is found in 5 to 30% of the general population [53]. Uric acid is associated with numerous renal and cardiovascular pathologies, being one of the consequences of these pathologies or linked to environmental factors responsible, among other things, for organ dysfunction. This is why, before considering a "lifelong" hypouricemic treatment "In order to avoid prescribing too early and to establish a definite indication, it is essential to take a holistic approach to the patient's health.

• Patient education

This is one of the fundamental points concerning the management of hyperuricemia, in patients who often present with several pathologies and comorbidities. For this reason, patients with chronic hyperuricemia must be made aware of the fact that it is associated with a higher risk of contracting numerous pathologies.Lifestyle changes such as a balanced diet, weight loss, exercise, smoking cessation and strict monitoring of associated diseases are essential in these patients, who often have one or more of the components of metabolic syndrome associated with them.

• Low-purine diet

High purine levels are found in the following foods [54]:

- Beef, pork or white meat (chicken, turkey);

- Fish (sardines, tuna) and seafood (shellfish);

- Some vegetables such as peas, lentils, asparagus, spinach, mushrooms
- All alcoholic beverages, especially beer;

- Giblets (gizzards and kidneys).

A purine-free diet can result in a 15-20% or 1.4 mg/dl reduction in uricemia. In contrast, a diet alone usually gives way to a high-carbohydrate, high-fat diet, with its effects on obesity, hypertriglyceridemia and other metabolic disorders[55].
On the other hand, several studies report that weight loss is positively correlated with a drop in uricemia, among other things, and increases renal clearance of uric acid.Patients with gout require a comprehensive, individualized dietary assessment.
This assessment is based on :

- weight loss,

- a low-calorie diet,

- a high-fiber diet,

- reduced alcohol consumption.

The first-line treatment of hyperuricemia is based on an appropriate diet, taking into account associated comorbidities.According to EULAR recommendations [58], hyperuricemic patients with more than two gout attacks per year, chronic arthropathy, tophi or radiological deformities related to gout should benefit from hypo-uricemic treatment.Since tissue urate levels are comparable to serum urate levels, the aim of treatment is to keep uricemia below 6 mg/dl.Because of the high risk of gout attacks on initiation, hypouricemic therapy should not be started within 15 days of a gout attack. It should be combined with gout prophylaxis for at least 3 to 6 months.

VI.2.3   Other drug treatments

- **Allopurinol**

Allopurinol, a purine xanthine oxidase inhibitor, is the historical first-line hypouricemic treatment. Uricemia must be monitored regularly on initiation to ensure target levels are reached, and should be considered for life.The maximum dose of allopurinol for patients with good renal function is 800mg/day. Doses should be increased every two weeks in 100mg increments, until a level of 6mg/dl (360 µmol/l) is reached. Dosage should also be adjusted according to the patient's age, renal status and tolerance.In addition to uricemia, clinical and biological monitoring is essential. Clinically, the focus is on skin and digestive tolerance; xanthic lithiasis is rare in cases of common gout. Biological monitoring includes twice-yearly checks of the CBC and liver enzymes (SGOT in particular). Intolerance to allopurinol manifests itself in the digestive tract, with nausea, vomiting and diarrhea in 5% of patients, without contraindicating treatment. In the skin, a pruritic erythematopapular or eczematous rash requires definitive discontinuation of treatment, as reintroduction would expose the patient to the risk of hypersensitivity syndrome (DRESS), a serious syndrome with a mortality rate of around 20%. [**59, 60**].

High initial doses of allopurinol (300 mg/d), the presence or onset of renal failure, and diuretic therapy all favor DRESS. Allopurinol exposes patients to the risk of neurological complications (peripheral neuropathy, Guillain-Barré syndrome) and, exceptionally, hematological accidents.Renal insufficiency may limit efficacy by imposing a dosage limitation. A study by Perez-Ruiz and associates showed that almost 50% of renal patients treated with allopurinol failed to reach the target uricemia of 360μmol/l [**61**].

Contraindications mainly concern drug interactions, especially with anti-vitamin K drugs (AVK) and chlorpropramide (hypoglycemic sulfonamide: risk of hypoglycemia, even more so in patients with renal insufficiency). Note the interaction between allopurinol and azathioprine, an immunosuppressant used mainly in organ transplant patients. Allopurinol blocks catabolism of purine anti-metabolics, increasing toxicity and induces a risk of hematological accident. The use of ampicillin on allopurinol also increases the frequency of skin rashes.

•**Febuxostat**

It is usually the second-line treatment in cases of contraindication (particularly moderate renal impairment) or intolerance to allopurinol. It is prescribed at a daily dose of 80 mg/d, and the target uricemia level (below 6 mg/dl) must be reached within 2 to 4 weeks of starting treatment. If not, the dose may be increased to 120 mg/d. Prophylactic treatment against gout attacks for 3 to 6 months is recommended, due to the increased risk of attacks at the start of hypouricemic treatment. The phase III APEX [**77**] and FACT [**62**] studies conducted in 2003 and 2004 demonstrated the superior efficacy of febuxostat 80-120 mg/d versus allopurinol 100-300 mg/d. In the febuxostat group, uricemia below 360 μmol/l was achieved in 48 and 65% of patients at 80 and 120 **mg/d**, compared with only 22% with allopurinol and 0% with placebo. The hypouricemic effect was achieved within two weeks and persisted throughout the study. In the subgroup of patients with renal insufficiency (Cl Cr>30 ml/min), at the allopurinol dose of 100 mg/day, the target uricemia level was not achieved. In the same group, target uricemia levels were 44% and 45% at febuxostat 80 and 120 mg/d respectively. The study therefore suggests superior efficacy compared with allopurinol, particularly in cases of moderate renal impairment where allopurinol doses need to be adapted. Due to predominantly hepatic metabolism, elevated transaminases have been observed. Diarrhea, headache, nausea and rash have also been reported. An incidence of cardiovascular events were observed in the febuxostat group in the APEX and FACT studies (1.3 vs. 0.3 events per 100 patient-years) and in the open-label extension phase (1.4 vs. 0.7 events per patient-year), without statistical significance, while the larger American CONFIRMS study found no cardiovascular events [63]. As a precaution, febuxostat should not be prescribed in cases of ischemic disease or congestive heart failure.

• **Uricosurics**

They lower uricemia by increasing urinary excretion of uric acid. Hence the risk of uric acid lithiasis, which must be prevented by abundant hydration and control of the urinary pH, which must be kept below 6, by alkalinizing the urine if necessary. They are therefore reserved for gout sufferers with no history of lithiasis and normal uricosuria.However, they are still available after a request for temporary use authorization from AFSSAPS, for patients intolerant to allopurinol and whose uricemia is not controlled by the probenicide.

• **Fenofibrate and Losartan**

They are a hypolipidemic and an antihypertensive, and are also uricosurics. Their efficacy is less than that of allopurinol and febuxostat, but they can be prescribed in gout patients preferentially for their indications.

• **Uricase**

Naturally present in most mammals, urate oxidase converts urate into allantoin. The gene encoding this enzyme has been inactivated in humans and apes, explaining physiological concentrations close to the solubility threshold in humans.

• **Rasburicase**

This is a recombinant aspergillar uricase, whose marketing authorization limits its use to the prevention of acute hyperuricemia in tumor lysis under chemotherapy. The hypouricemic effect is powerful, but numerous side effects have been reported (allergic reactions, development of antibodies directed against uricase) and its half-life is very short (less than 24h). This severely limits its use.

• **Pegloticase**

This is a pegylated recombinant porcine uricase administered intravenously every 2 weeks. It was recently approved by the FDA for the treatment of gout refractory to conventional hypo-uricemics. It is not marketed in France. A pharmacokinetic study [64] showed that a single intravenous administration of 4 to 12 mg of pegloticase ensured significant uricase activity in patients' serum for 21 days. Uricemia decreased dramatically 24 to 72 hours after infusion. A phase II trial [65] was conducted on 41 patients with severe and refractory gout. They received pegloticase at various administration schedules, for 12 to 14 weeks. Mean uricemia fell below 360 µmol/l within 6 h for all doses. The optimal dose was 8 mg every 2 weeks. Anti-pegloticase antibodies were observed in 31 of 41 patients, associated with a decreased half-life of the molecule. Gout attacks were triggered in 88% of patients following administration of pegloticase. Two 6-month Phase III studies randomized in 3 arms (pegloticase 8 mg every 2 weeks, every 4 weeks or placebo) 212 patients with refractory gout [66]. All received colchicine and/or cortisone prior to infusion. Results showed a clear reduction in uricemia in patients on pegloticase (47 and 38% responders, responders being defined as having uricemia < 360 µmol/l for 80% of the last 3 months of the study, versus 0 in the placebo arm). At least one tophus disappeared in 45% and 26% of patients on pegloticase, versus 8% on placebo. On the other hand, there was an increase in gouty attacks during the first 3 months after introduction of pegloticase (75% and 81% versus 53% on placebo). On the other hand, there was a reduction in gouty attacks in the last 3 months of the study (41% and 57% versus 67% on placebo).Reported adverse events are mainly related to allergic reactions, sometimes severe. Antibodies directed against uricase were developed in 59% of patients, leading to a loss of treatment efficacy (with uricemia rising above 360 µmol/l).Pegloticase therefore requires close monitoring in view of its allergic side effects. It is also contraindicated in cases of G6PD deficiency.

• Ulodesin (BCX4208)

It is a purine phosphorylase inhibitor acting upstream of xanthine oxidase inhibitors. It can prevent the formation of uric acid.A phase II study was carried out on 278 gouty patients with inclusion criteria of uricemia > 360 µmol/l despite taking 300 mg/day of allopurinol. They were randomized into 5 arms (ulodesin 5, 10, 20 or 40 mg/d, or placebo). Follow-up lasted 12 weeks.The rate of adverse events was comparable in the 5 groups. A dose-dependent decrease in lymphocyte count was noted. However, the rate remained stable during follow-up, but led to 15 discontinuations in the 2 arms receiving the highest doses. The results show that the target uricemia level is reached in 36% to 41% of patients in the ulodesine groups, compared with 22% in the placebo group. This molecule could become a useful adjunct in patients refractory to allopurinol **[67]**.

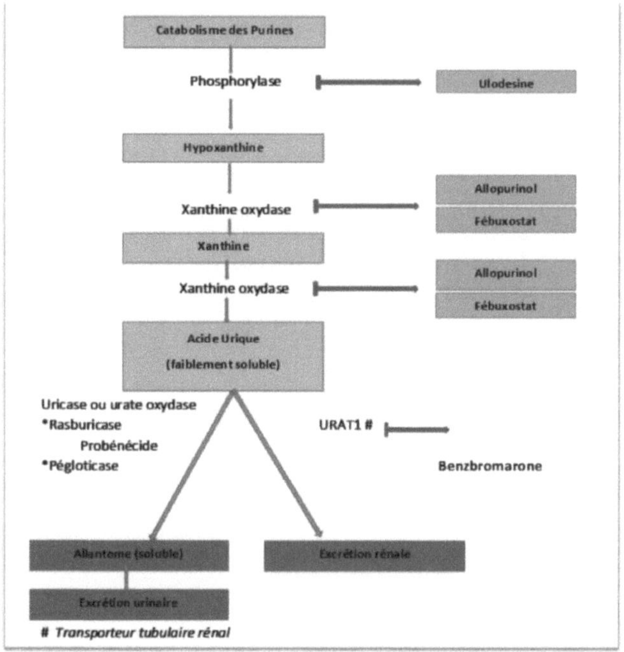

Figure 5: Uric acid formation and mechanism of action of hypouricemic treatments **[87].**

VI.3 Indications [69]

VI.3.1 Isolated hyperuricemia :

Authors currently agree that isolated hyperuricemia should not be treated systematically, especially as the side effects of hypo-uricemic drugs entail certain serious risks. Hygienic and dietary measures should be preferred. The only exception is the occurrence of major iatrogenic hyperuricemia, notably in the treatment of hematological malignancies with cytolytics.

VI.3.2 Drop

There are two alternatives: some authors start hypo-uricaemic treatment as soon as the first gout attack occurs, if hyperuricaemia is present.Others, perhaps the most numerous, wait until several attacks have occurred before initiating hypo-uremic treatment if the symptoms are disabling. In cases of chronic gout and renal manifestations, hypo-uricemic treatment is imperative.

CONCLUSION

Unlike some African and Western countries, studies of gout are still rare in Senegal.

REFERENCES

[1] Pierre Lafforgue, Virginie Legré.

Diseases and Major Syndromes, Microcrystalline arthropathies

Module Pluridisciplinaire n° 13 Rhumatologie, Chirurgie Orthopédique,

Chirurgie Infantile, Faculté de Médecine de Marseille DCEM 3, 2005

[2] Tony R.Merriman, NicolaDalbeth. Genetic basis of hyperuricemia and gout.
Revue du rhumatisme monographies 77(2010)328-334 329.

[3] Puig JG, Torres RJ.

Hypoxanthine-guanine phosophoribosyltransferase (HGPRT) deficiency: Lesch-Nyhan syndrome.

Orphanet J Rare Dis 2007;2:48

[4] Sébastien Faure.

Anti-gout. Fiche pharmacothérapeutique pratique. Actualités pharmaceutiques. n°
495.April 2010

[5] Pascal Richette, Thomas Bardin.

Gout, Vol 375 January 23, 2010

[6] Annemans L

Spaepen E, Gaskin M, Bonnemaire M, Malier V, Gilbert T, et al. Gout in the
UK and Germany: prevalence, comorbidities and management in general practice
2000-2005. Ann Rheum Dis. Jul 2008;67(7):960-6.

[7] LENNANE GA, ROSE BS, ISDALE IC. Gout in the Maori. Ann Rheum
Dis. June 1960;19:120-5.

[8] Klemp P, Stansfield SA, Castle B, Robertson MC. Gout is on the increase in
New Zealand. Ann Rheum Dis. Jan 1997;56(1):22-6.

[9] Wallace KL, Riedel AA, Joseph-Ridge N, Wortmann R. Increasing
prevalence of gout and hyperuricemia over 10 years among older adults in a
managed care population. J Rheumatol. August 2004;31(8):1582-7.

[10] Lawrence RC, Helmick CG, Arnett FC, Deyo RA, Felson DT, Giannini
EH, et al. Estimates of the prevalence of arthritis and selected musculoskeletal

disorders in the United States. Arthritis Rheum. May 1998;41(5):778-99.

[11] Currie WJ. Prevalence and incidence of the diagnosis of gout in Great Britain. Ann Rheum Dis. Apr 1979;38(2):101-6.

[12] Kuo C-F, Grainge MJ, Mallen C, Zhang W, Doherty M. Rising burden of gout in the UK but continuing suboptimal management: a nationwide population study. Ann Rheum Dis. Apr 2015;74(4):661-7

[13] Arromdee E, Michet CJ, Crowson CS, O'Fallon WM, Gabriel SE. Epidemiology of gout: is the incidence rising? J Rheumatol. nov 2002;29(11):24036.

[14] Elliot AJ, Cross KW, Fleming DM. Seasonality and trends in the incidence and prevalence of gout in England and Wales 1994-2007. Ann Rheum Dis. Nov 2009;68(11):1728-33.

[15] Zhang W, Doherty M, Pascual E, Bardin T, Barskova V, Conaghan P, et al. EULAR evidence based recommendations for gout. Part I: Diagnosis. Report of a task force of the Standing Committee for International Clinical Studies Including Therapeutics (ESCISIT). Ann Rheum Dis. Oct 2006;65(10):1301-11.

[16] Ea H-K. [Mechanisms of gout inflammation]. Presse Médicale Paris Fr 1983. sept 2011;40(9 Pt 1):836-43.

[17] Joosten LAB, Netea MG, Mylona E, Koenders MI, Malireddi RKS, Oosting M, et al. Engagement of fatty acids with Toll-like receptor 2 drives interleukin-1β production via the ASC/caspase 1 pathway in monosodium urate monohydrate crystal-induced gouty arthritis. Arthritis Rheum. nov 2010;62(11):3237-48.

[18] Dalbeth N, Haskard DO. Mechanisms of inflammation in gout. Rheumatol Oxf Engl. Sept 2005;44(9):1090-6.

[19] Lioté F, Ea H-K. Recent developments in crystal-induced inflammation pathogenesis and management. Curr Rheumatol Rep. June 2007;9(3):243-50.

[20] Lioté F, Prudhommeaux F, Schiltz C, Champy R, Herbelin A, Ortiz-Bravo E,et al. Inhibition and prevention of monosodium urate monohydrate crystal-induced acute inflammation in vivo by transforming growth factor beta1. Arthritis Rheum. July 1996;39(7):1192-8.

[21] Shi Y, Mucsi AD, Ng G. Monosodium urate crystals in inflammation and immunity. Immunol Rev. Jan 2010;233(1):203-17.

[22] Pétrilli V, Martinon F. The inflammasome, autoinflammatory diseases, and gout. Jt Bone Spine Rev Rhum. Dec 2007;74(6):571-6.

[23] Martinon F. Mechanisms of uric acid crystal-mediated autoinflammation. Immunol Rev. Jan 2010;233(1):218-32

[24] Dalbeth N, Pool B, Gamble GD, Smith T, Callon KE, McQueen FM, et al. Cellular characterization of the gouty tophus: a quantitative analysis. Arthritis Rheum. May 2010;62(5):1549-56.

[25] Dalbeth N, Smith T, Nicolson B, Clark B, Callon K, Naot D, et al. Enhanced osteoclastogenesis in patients with tophaceous gout: urate crystals promote osteoclast development through interactions with stromal cells. Arthritis Rheum. June 2008;58(6):1854-65.

[26] Bouchard L, de Médicis R, Lussier A, Naccache PH, Poubelle PE. Inflammatory microcrystals alter the functional phenotype of human osteoblast-like cells in vitro: synergism with IL-1 to overexpress cyclooxygenase-2. J Immunol Baltim Md 1950. May 15, 2002;168(10):5310-7.

[27] Zhang W, Doherty M, Bardin T, Pascual E, Barskova V, Conaghan P, et al. EULAR evidence based recommendations for gout. Part II: Management. Report of a task force of the EULAR Standing Committee for International Clinical Studies Including Therapeutics (ESCISIT). Ann Rheum Dis. Oct 2006;65(10):1312-24.

[28] **Hang Korng.** From hyperuricemia to gout: pathophysiology / Revue du Rhumatisme 78 (2011) S103-S108

[29] **J. Taillandier, M. Alemanni, C. Trivalle, M. Harboun.** Prevalence of hyperuricemia in elderly women. Revue du Rhumatisme 74 (2007) 1039-1208

[30] **Alexander So, Nathalie Busso.** Gout news in 2012. Revue du Rhumatisme 79S (2012) A22-A26

[31] Graessler J, Graessler A, Unger S, Kopprasch S, Tausche A-K, Kuhlisch E, et

al. Association of the human urate transporter 1 with reduced renal uric acid excretion and hyperuricemia in a German Caucasian population. Arthritis Rheum. Jan 2006;54(1):292-300.

[32] Dehghan A, Köttgen A, Yang Q, Hwang S-J, Kao WL, Rivadeneira F, et al. Association of three genetic loci with uric acid concentration and risk of gout: a genome-wide association study. Lancet. Dec 6, 2008;372(9654):1953-61.

[33] Gérard Chalès. From hyperuricemia to gout: epidemiology of gout. Revue du Rhumatisme 78 (2011) S109-S115

[34] **Sylvie Rozenberg**, La goutte médicamenteuse, Revue du Rhumatisme 74,150-152. 2007

[35] Choi HK, Ford ES, Li C, Curhan G. Prevalence of the metabolic syndrome in patients with gout: the Third National Health and Nutrition Examination Survey. Arthritis Rheum. Feb 15, 2007;57(1):109-15.

[36] Richette P, Bardin T. Gout. Lancet. 23 Jan 2010;375(9711):318-28.

[37] Hull RG. Polyarticular gout. Lancet. May 20, 1989;1(8647):1142.

[38] Khanna D, Fitzgerald JD, Khanna PP, Bae S, Singh MK, Neogi T, et al. 2012 American College of Rheumatology guidelines for management of gout. Part 1: systematic nonpharmacologic and pharmacologic therapeutic approaches to hyperuricemia. Arthritis Care Res. Oct 2012;64(10):1431-46.

[39] Khanna D, Khanna PP, Fitzgerald JD, Singh MK, Bae S, Neogi T, et al. 2012 American College of Rheumatology guidelines for management of gout. Part 2: therapy and antiinflammatory prophylaxis of acute gouty arthritis. Arthritis Care Res. Oct 2012;64(10):1447-61.

[40] Janssens HJEM, Janssen M, van de Lisdonk EH, van Riel PLCM, van Weel C. Use of oral prednisolone or naproxen for the treatment of gout arthritis: a double- blind, randomised equivalence trial. Lancet. May 31, 2008;371(9627):1854-60.

[41] Laine L, White WB, Rostom A, Hochberg M. COX-2 selective inhibitors in the treatment of osteoarthritis. Semin Arthritis Rheum. Dec 2008;38(3):165-87.

[42] Jordan KM, Cameron JS, Snaith M, Zhang W, Doherty M, Seckl J, et al. British Society for Rheumatology and British Health Professionals in Rheumatology guideline for the management of gout. Rheumatol Oxf Engl. August 2007;46(8):1372-4.

[43] Rubin BR, Burton R, Navarra S, Antigua J, Londoño J, Pryhuber KG, et al. Efficacy and safety profile of treatment with etoricoxib 120 mg once daily compared with indomethacin 50 mg three times daily in acute gout: a randomized controlled trial. Arthritis Rheum. Feb 2004;50(2):598-606.

[44] Willburger RE, Mysler E, Derbot J, Jung T, Thurston H, Kreiss A, et al. Lumiracoxib 400 mg once daily is comparable to indomethacin 50 mg three times daily for the treatment of acute flares of gout. Rheumatol Oxf Engl. July 2007;46(7):1126-32.

[45] Schumacher HR, Berger MF, Li-Yu J, Perez-Ruiz F, Burgos-Vargas R, Li C. Efficacy and tolerability of celecoxib in the treatment of acute gouty arthritis: a randomized controlled trial. J Rheumatol. Sept 2012;39(9):1859-66.

[46] Schlesinger N, Schumacher R, Catton M, Maxwell L. Colchicine for acute gout. Cochrane Database Syst Rev. 2006;(4):CD006190.

[47] Terkeltaub RA. Colchicine update: 2008. Semin Arthritis Rheum. June 2009;38(6):411-9.

[48] Nuki G. Colchicine: its mechanism of action and efficacy in crystal-induced inflammation. Curr Rheumatol Rep. July 2008;10(3):218-27.

[49] Janssens HJEM, Lucassen PLBJ, Van de Laar FA, Janssen M, Van de Lisdonk EH. Systemic corticosteroids for acute gout. Cochrane Database Syst Rev. 2008;(2):CD005521.

[50] Gaffo AL, Saag KG. Are glucocorticoids equivalent to NSAIDs for the treatment of gout flares? Nat Clin Pract Rheumatol. Jan 2009;5(1):12-3.

[51] Schlesinger N, Mysler E, Lin H-Y, De Meulemeester M, Rovensky J, Arulmani U, et al. Canakinumab reduces the risk of acute gouty arthritis flares during initiation of allopurinol treatment: results of a double-blind, randomised study. Ann Rheum Dis. Jul 2011;70(7):1264-71.

[52] Schumacher HR Jr, Evans RR, Saag KG, Clower J, Jennings W, Weinstein SP, et al. Rilonacept (interleukin-1 trap) for prevention of gout flares during initiation of uric acidlowering therapy: results from a phase III randomized, double-blind, placebo-controlled, confirmatory efficacy study. Arthritis Care Res. Oct 2012;64(10):1462-70.

[53] Rott KT, Agudelo CA. Gout. JAMA J Am Med Assoc. June 4, 2003;289(21):2857-60.

[54] Wolfram G, Colling M. [Total purine content in selected foods]. Z Für Ernährungswissenschaft. Dec 1987;26(4):205-13.

[55] Maclachlan MJ, Rodnan GP. Effect of food, fast and alcohol on serum uric acid and acute attacks of gout. Am J Med. Jan 1967;42(1):38-57.

[56] Gibson T, Rodgers AV, Simmonds HA, Court-Brown F, Todd E, Meilton V. A controlled study of diet in patients with gout. Ann Rheum Dis. Apr 1983;42(2):123-7.

[57] Dessein PH, Shipton EA, Stanwix AE, Joffe BI, Ramokgadi J. Beneficial effects of weight loss associated with moderate calorie/carbohydrate restriction, and increased proportional intake of protein and unsaturated fat on serum urate and lipoprotein levels in gout: a pilot study. Ann Rheum Dis. Jul 2000;59(7):539-43.

[58] Hamburger M, Baraf HSB, Adamson TC 3rd, Basile J, Bass L, Cole B, et al. 2011 Recommendations for the diagnosis and management of gout and hyperuricemia. Postgrad Med. nov 2011;123(6 Suppl 1):3-36.

[59] Markel A. Allopurinol-induced DRESS syndrome. Isr Med Assoc J IMAJ. Oct 2005;7(10):656-60.

[60] Roujeau J-C. Clinical heterogeneity of drug hypersensitivity. Toxicology. 15 Apr 2005;209(2):123-9.

[61] Perez-Ruiz F, Alonso-Ruiz A, Calabozo M, Herrero-Beites A, García-Erauskin G, RuizLucea E. Efficacy of allopurinol and benzbromarone for the control of hyperuricaemia. A pathogenic approach to the treatment of primary chronic gout. Ann Rheum Dis. Sept 1998;57(9):545-9.

[62] Becker MA, Schumacher HR Jr, Wortmann RL, MacDonald PA, Eustace D, Palo WA, et al. Febuxostat compared with allopurinol in patients with hyperuricemia and gout. N Engl J Med. Dec 8, 2005;353(23):2450-61.

[63] Becker MA, Schumacher HR, Espinoza LR, Wells AF, MacDonald P, Lloyd E, et al. The urate-lowering efficacy and safety of febuxostat in the treatment of the hyperuricemia of gout: the CONFIRMS trial. Arthritis Res Ther. 2010;12(2):R63.

[64] Sundy JS, Ganson NJ, Kelly SJ, Scarlett EL, Rehrig CD, Huang W, et al. Pharmacokinetics and pharmacodynamics of intravenous PEGylated recombinant mammalian urate oxidase in patients with refractory gout. Arthritis Rheum. March 2007;56(3):1021-8.

[65] Sherman MR, Saifer MGP, Perez-Ruiz F. PEG-uricase in the management of treatmentresistant gout and hyperuricemia. Adv Drug Deliv Rev. Jan 3, 2008;60(1):59-68.

[66] Schlesinger N, Yasothan U, Kirkpatrick P. Pegloticase. Nat Rev Drug Discov. Jan 2011;10(1):17-8.

[67] Crittenden DB, Pillinger MH. New therapies for gout. Annu Rev Med. 2013;64:325-37.

[68] P.Richette, T.Bardin.la lettre du Rhumatologue N°384-September 2012.

[69] C.Sylla.l'approche steps wise de la goutte dans le service de Rhumatologie au CHU de Point G à Bamako; thèse medecine,2009-2010.

[70] M Mijiyawa, M Bouglouga Hyperuricemie et Goutte en zone intertropicale Rev Rhum 2003; 70: 152-156

[71] **Moustafa Mijiyawa, Owonayo Oniankitan :**Risk factors for gout in Togolese patients ;Revue du rhumatisme Volume 67, n° 8 pages 621-626 (october 2000)

[72] M Mijiyawa, O Oniankita Risk factors for gout in Togolese patients. Rev Rhum 2000; 67: 621-6.

[73] M C Boisier Goutte : in décision en Rhumatologie Edition Viget Paris 1996 ; 257-266

[74] T Bardin Arthropathies microcristallines du sujet âgé. Polyarthritis and inflammatory rheumatism in the elderly Rev Rhum 2003; 70: 180-199

[75] "Gout crisis" Rev Prescrire 2017; 37 (404): 442-445. Frédéric Lioté*, Thomas Bardin: **Revue du Rhumatisme 74 (2007) 160 -167 Traitement de la goutte ;** Fédération de rhumatologie, pôle locomoteur, center Viggo-Petersen, hôpital Lariboisière, APHP, 2, rue Ambroise-Paré, 75010 Paris, France.

[76] https://fr.wikipedia.org/wiki/Goutte_(illness)

[77] https://www.planetesante.ch/Magazine/Autour-de-la-disease/Rheumatism/Gout-a-rheumatism-in-full-expansion

[78] https://docplayer.fr/14033272-Imagerie-populaire-de-la-goutte-maladie- old-fashioned-unscientific-19th-century-she-was-responsible-for-every-evil-drop-remontee.html

[79] Guide pratique de rhumatologie $2nd$ edition, Bernard Mazière, Alain Cantagrel, Michel Laroche, Arnaud Constantin, Masson 2002, p66-73.

[80] COFER, knowledge and practice in rheumatology. Masson Editeur, June 2004, Tournai-Belgium

[81] G Kaplan, A Prier, Ph Vinceneux Rhumatologie pour le praticien ; SIMEP, Paris, 1990.

[82] F Leclereq, M G Malaise. Gout Rev Med 2004; 59: 274-280

[83] M Hilliquin La goutte : principales manifestations Concours Médical 2004 ; 126 : 1589-1592

[84] P Guggenbuhi, Y Pawlostsky, G Chalès What's new in gout in 2002. Rev Rhum; 286: 17-26

[85] Buchard Rhumatismes iatrogènes Rev Med Suisse Romande 2004 ; 124 : 551-555

[86] https://www.google.com/search?q=goutte+chronic&sxsrf=ACYBGNT wn_oTkSw2kpdRBp9aiR4mL-KZ8w:1575736993823&source=lnms&tbm=isch&sa=X&ved=2ahUKEwj6vZre_

aPmAhUsAWMBHaeqAW0Q_AUoAXoECBAQAw&biw=1366&bih=625#imgd
ii=V-5rKPe16lUgJM:&imgrc=9n1pYmyrmOBqVM:

[87] (Nouvelles données dans la goutte, G. Moutarde, la lettre du
Rhumatologue, supplement to n°390, March 2013, p17).

CONTENTS

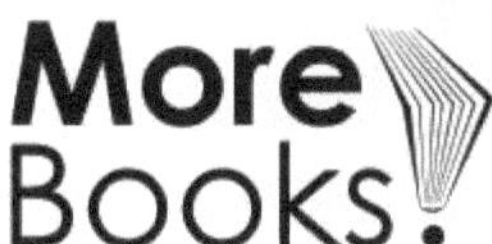

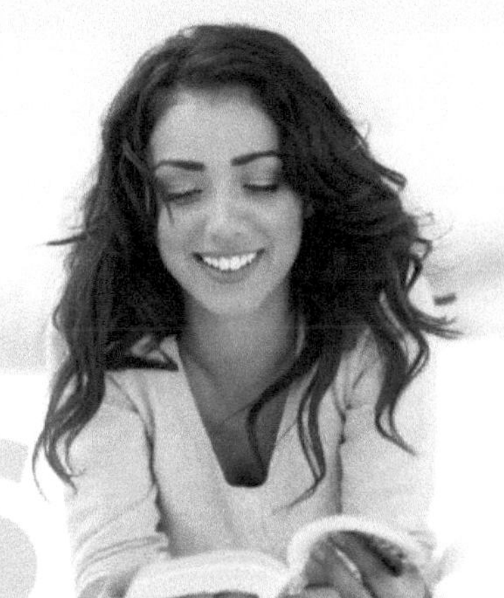

I want morebooks!

Buy your books fast and straightforward online - at one of world's fastest growing online book stores! Environmentally sound due to Print-on-Demand technologies.

Buy your books online at
www.morebooks.shop

Kaufen Sie Ihre Bücher schnell und unkompliziert online – auf einer der am schnellsten wachsenden Buchhandelsplattformen weltweit! Dank Print-On-Demand umwelt- und ressourcenschonend produzi ert.

Bücher schneller online kaufen
www.morebooks.shop

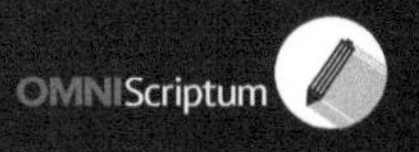

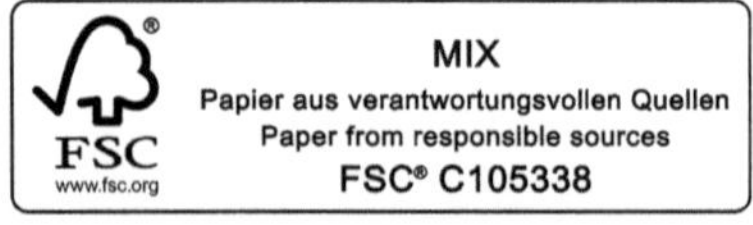

Printed by Books on Demand GmbH, Norderstedt / Germany